39 All-natural Breast Cancer Juice Recipes:

The Most Effective Way to Treat and Prevent Breast Cancer through Organic Ingredients

By

Joe Correa CSN

COPYRIGHT

This publication is designed to provide accurate and authoritative information in regard to the subject matter covered. It is sold with the understanding that neither the author nor the publisher is engaged in rendering medical advice. If medical advice or assistance is needed, consult with a doctor. This book is considered a guide and should not be used in any way detrimental to your health. Consult with a physician before starting this nutritional plan to make sure it's right for you.

ACKNOWLEDGEMENTS

This book is dedicated to my friends and family that have had mild or serious illnesses so that you may find a solution and make the necessary changes in your life.

39 All-natural Breast Cancer Juice Recipes:

The Most Effective Way to Treat and Prevent Breast Cancer through Organic Ingredients

By

Joe Correa CSN

CONTENTS

ABOUT THE AUTHOR

After years of Research, I honestly believe in the positive effects that proper nutrition can have over the body and mind. My knowledge and experience has helped me live healthier throughout the years and which I have shared with family and friends. The more you know about eating and drinking healthier, the sooner you will want to change your life and eating habits.

Nutrition is a key part in the process of being healthy and living longer so get started today. The first step is the most important and the most significant.

INTRODUCTION

39 All-natural Breast Cancer Juice Recipes: The Most Effective Way to Treat and Prevent Breast Cancer through Organic Ingredients

By Joe Correa CSN

Breast cancer is the most common form of cancer among women and it is extremely important to learn the facts about the biology of breast tissue and the symptoms of this terrible disease.

A women's breasts are made of glands that produce milk for breastfeeding, fat, and connective tissue. This tissue develops during puberty with normal cell growth over the years.

Just like any other type of cancer, breast cancer starts with abnormal and uncontrollable cell growth. The cause of this process is unknown, but fortunately, the symptoms are quite obvious and can be spotted quickly. It's crucial to notice the earliest symptoms which include:

-   A change in the skin texture around the nipple area. These changes include unusual nipple tenderness or thickening of tissue. These abnormalities are usually followed by an enlargement of pores that patients describe as an orange peel. In these cases, the skin or the nipple becomes red and changes its natural color.

- A newly formed lump in the breast area. It's important to mention that all lumps require your attention and should be examined by a healthcare professional.
- Abnormal change in the size of one or both breasts. If you notice some unexplained growth or swelling of the breast tissue, it's important to visit your doctor. The same goes for unnatural shrinkage of one or both breasts.
- An unexplained milky discharge from one or both breast can also mean an early development of breast cancer and should be examined by your doctor.

Fortunately, new medical treatments have dramatically improved the survival rate in women suffering from breast cancer.

I sincerely hope this book will increase your awareness of this serious disease and teach you how some simple lifestyle changes can dramatically improve your health and prevent any life-threatening conditions.

In this book, you will find amazingly delicious juice recipes that are based on super-healthy ingredients which are proven to boost up the immune system and fight off different types of cancer, including breast cancer. These juices are extremely easy to make and won't take much of your time. When combined with a regular self-exam, these foods are the key to preventing this horrible disease.

Stay happy and healthy with these great breast cancer preventing juices!

39 ALL-NATURAL BREAST CANCER JUICE RECIPES: THE MOST EFFECTIVE WAY TO TREAT AND PREVENT BREAST CANCER THROUGH ORGANIC INGREDIENTS

1.   Zucchini Celery Juice

Ingredients:

1 large zucchini, chopped

1 cup of celery, chopped

2 cups of Brussels sprouts, halved

1 cup of green cabbage, torn

¼ tsp of Himalayan salt

2 oz of water

Preparation:

Peel the zucchini and cut in half. Scoop out the seeds and chop into small pieces. Set aside.

Wash the celery and cut into small pieces. Set aside.

Wash the Brussels sprouts and trim off the outer leaves. Cut in half and set aside.

Wash the cabbage thoroughly under cold running water. Drain and torn with hands. Set aside.

Now, combine, zucchini, celery, Brussel sprouts, and cabbage in a juicer and process until juiced. Transfer to serving glasses and stir in the Himalayan salt and water.

Add few ice cubes or refrigerate before serving.

Enjoy!

Nutritional information per serving: Kcal: 115, Protein: 11.7g, Carbs: 33.9g, Fats: 1.8g

2.   Celery Grapefruit Juice

Ingredients:

1 cup of celery, chopped

1 whole grapefruit, peeled

2 large carrots, chunked

1 small Golden Delicious apple, cored and chopped

¼ tsp of cinnamon, ground

Preparation:

Wash the celery and cut into small pieces. Fill the measuring cup and reserve the rest in the refrigerator.

Peel the grapefruit and divide into wedges. Cut each wedge in half and set aside.

Wash and peel the carrots. Cut into small chunks and set aside.

Wash the apple and cut lengthwise in half. Remove the core and cut into bite-sized pieces. Set aside.

Now, combine carrots, celery, grapefruit, and apple in a juicer and process until well juiced. Transfer to a serving glass and stir in the cinnamon.

Add some crushed ice and serve immediately.

Enjoy!

Nutritional information per serving: Kcal: 203, Protein: 4.3g, Carbs: 60.6g, Fats: 1.1g

3.   Basil Cucumber Juice

Ingredients:

1 cup of basil, torn

1 cup of cucumber, sliced

1 medium-sized artichoke, chopped

1 whole lime, peeled

2 oz of water

Preparation:

Wash the basil thoroughly under cold running water. Drain and torn into small pieces. Set aside.

Wash the cucumber and cut into thin slices. Fill the measuring cup and reserve the rest in the refrigerator.

Trim off the outer leaves of the artichoke. Wash it and chop into small pieces. Set aside.

Peel the lime and cut lengthwise in half. Set aside.

Now, combine artichoke, basil, cucumber, and lime in a juicer and process until juiced. Transfer to a serving glass and stir in the water.

Refrigerate for 5 minutes before serving.

Nutrition information per serving: Kcal: 53, Protein: 5.5g, Carbs: 19.6g, Fats: 0.4g

4.   Asparagus Collard Green Juice

Ingredients:

1 medium-sized tomato, chopped

1 cup of asparagus, trimmed and chopped

1 cup of collard greens, torn

1 cup of spinach, torn

¼ tsp salt

1 rosemary sprig

Preparation:

Wash the asparagus and trim off the woody ends. Cut into small pieces and fill the measuring cup. Set aside.

Combine collard greens and spinach in a large colander. Wash under cold running water and drain. Torn into small pieces and set aside.

Wash the tomato and place it in a small bowl. Cut into small pieces and reserve the tomato juice while cutting. Set aside.

Now, combine asparagus, collard greens, tomato, and spinach in a juicer and process until juiced. Transfer to a serving glass and stir in the reserve tomato juice and salt. Sprinkle with rosemary.

You can add some basil for some extra taste, but it's optional.

Serve immediately.

Nutritional information per serving: Kcal: 66, Protein: 11.2g, Carbs: 19.6g, Fats: 1.5g

5.   Kiwi Apple Juice

Ingredients:

1 whole kiwi, peeled

1 small Grany Smith's apple, cored

1 cup of mango, chopped

1 small ginger knob, peeled

2 oz of coconut water

Preparation:

Peel the kiwi and cut lengthwise in half. Set aside.

Wash the apple and cut lengthwise in half. Remove the core and cut into small pieces. Set aside.

Peel the mango and cut into small pieces. Fill the measuring cup and reserve the rest for later.

Peel the ginger knob and cut into small pieces. Set aside.

Now, combine mango, kiwi, apple, and ginger in a juicer and process until juiced. Transfer to a serving glass and stir in the coconut water. Add some crushed ice and serve immediately.

Enjoy!

Nutrition information per serving: Kcal: 196, Protein: 2.8g, Carbs: 55.5g, Fats: 1.3g

6.   Celery Plum Juice

Ingredients:

1 cup of celery, chopped

1 whole plum, pitted and chopped

1 small Golden Delicious apple, cored

1 cup of cherries

¼ tsp of cinnamon, ground

2 tbsp of coconut water

Preparation:

Wash and trim off the celery. Chop into small pieces and set aside.

Wash the plum and cut in half. Remove the pit and chop into small pieces. Set aside.

Wash the apple and cut lengthwise in half. Remove the core and cut into bite-sized pieces. Set aside.

Wash the cherries using a colander. Drain and cut each in half. Remove the pits and set aside.

Now, combine celery, plum, apple, cherries, in a juicer and

process until juiced. Transfer to a serving glass and stir in the cinnamon and coconut water.

Add some crushed ice and serve immediately.

Nutritional information per serving: Kcal: 182, Protein: 3.1g, Carbs: 52.7g, Fats: 0.8g

7.   Squash Zucchini Juice

Ingredients:

1 cup of butternut squash, chopped

1 cup of crookneck squash, chopped

1 large zucchini

1 cup of pumpkin, chopped

1 large carrot

¼ tsp of nutmeg, ground

¼ tsp of salt

2 oz of water

Preparation:

Peel the butternut squash and remove the seeds using a spoon. Cut into small cubes and reserve the rest of the squash for some other recipe. Wrap in a plastic foil and refrigerate.

Wash the crookneck squash and cut in half. Scoop out the seeds using a spoon. Cut into small chunks and set aside. Reserve the rest for another juice.

Peel the zucchini and cut in lengthwise in half. Scrap out the seeds and cut into chunks. Set aside.

Peel the pumpkin and cut in half. Scoop out the seeds using a spoon. Cut one large wedge and peel it. Cut into small chunks and set aside. Reserve the rest for later.

Wash the carrot and cut into thick slices. Set aside.

Now, process butternut squash, crookneck squash, zucchini, pumpkin, and carrot in a juicer.

Transfer to serving glasses and stir in the Himalayan salt and water. Refrigerate for 5 minutes before serving.

Enjoy!

Nutritional information per serving: Kcal: 163, Protein: 8.4g, Carbs: 45.8g, Fats: 1.8g

8.   Carrot Pepper Juice

Ingredients:

1 large carrot

1 large red bell pepper

1 cup of cauliflower, chopped

1 large orange

1 cup of fresh kale, torn

¼ tsp of Himalayan salt

3 oz of water

Preparation:

Wash the carrot and cut into thick slices. Set aside.

Wash the red bell pepper and cut in half. Remove the seeds and cut in small pieces. Set aside.

Trim off the outer leaves of a cauliflower. Wash it and cut into small pieces and fill the measuring cup. Reserve the rest in the refrigerator.

Peel the orange and divide into wedges. Set aside.

Wash the kale thoroughly and torn with hands. Set aside.

Now, process carrot, red bell pepper, cauliflower, orange, and kale in a juicer. Transfer to serving glasses and stir in the salt and water.

Refrigerate for 5 minutes before serving.

Enjoy!

Nutritional information per serving: Kcal: 169, Protein: 8.9g, Carbs: 49.6g, Fats: 1.8g

9.   Apple Cucumber Juice

Ingredients:

1 large Granny Smith apple

1 large cucumber

1 large fennel

1 rosemary sprig

¼ tsp of Himalayan salt

2 oz of water

Preparation:

Wash the apple and remove the core. Cut into bite-sized pieces and set aside.

Wash the cucumber and cut into thick pieces. Set aside.

Wash the fennel bulb and trim off the wilted outer layers. Cut into small chunks and set aside.

Now, process fennel, apple, and cucumber in a juicer. Transfer to serving glasses and stir in the Himalayan salt and water. Sprinkle with rosemary and refrigerate for 10 minutes before serving.

Enjoy!

Nutritional information per serving: Kcal: 179, Protein: 5.7g, Carbs: 56g, Fats: 1.2g

10.   Carrot Apple Juice

Ingredients:

3 large carrots

1 large green apple, cored

1 large orange

1 cup of watermelon, diced

1 cup of green grapes

1 small ginger root knob, 1-inch

Preparation:

Wash the carrots and cut into thick slices. Set aside.

Wash the apple and remove the core. Cut into bite-sized pieces and set aside.

Peel the orange and divide into wedges. Set aside.

Cut the watermelon lengthwise. For one cup, you will need about 1 large wedge. Peel and cut into chunks. Remove the seeds and set aside. Reserve the rest of the melon for some other juices.

Wash the grapes under cold running water. Drain and set aside.

Peel the ginger root knob and set aside.

Now, combine carrots, apple, orange, watermelon, grapes, and ginger in a juicer and process until juiced.

Transfer to serving glasses and add some ice before serving.

Enjoy!

Nutritional information per serving: Kcal: 335, Protein: 6.2g, Carbs: 98g, Fats: 1.7g

11.   Leek Lime Juice

Ingredients:

1 whole leek, chopped

1 whole lime, peeled

1 large orange, peeled

1 small green apple, cored

Preparation:

Wash the leek and chop into small pieces. Set aside.

Peel the lemon and lime. Cut each fruit lengthwise in half and set aside.

Peel the orange and divide into wedges. Cut each wedge in half and set aside.

Wash the apple and cut in half. Remove the core and cut into small pieces. Set aside.

Now, combine lemon, leek, lime, orange, and apple in a juicer and process until juiced. Transfer to a serving glass and refrigerate for 15 minutes before serving.

Enjoy!

Nutrition information per serving: Kcal: 205, Protein: 4.5g, Carbs: 62.9g, Fats: 0.9g

12. Pineapple Raspberry Juice

Ingredients:

1 cup of pineapple chunks

1 cup of raspberries

1 large mango

1 large orange

2 oz of coconut water

Preparation:

Cut the top of a pineapple and peel it using a sharp knife. Cut into small chunks. Reserve the rest of the pineapple in a refrigerator.

Place the raspberries in a colander and wash under cold running water. Drain and set aside.

Wash the mango and cut into bite-sized pieces. Set aside.

Peel the orange and divide into wedges. Set aside.

Now, combine, pineapple, raspberries, mango, and orange in a juicer and process until juiced. Transfer to serving glasses and stir in the coconut water.

Add some ice and serve immediately!

Nutritional information per serving: Kcal: 353, Protein: 6.8, Carbs: 108g, Fats: 2.5g

13.   Blackberry Kiwi Juice

Ingredients:

1 cup of blackberries

2 whole kiwis, peeled

1 cup of cantaloupe, chopped

1 small green apple, cored

¼ tsp of ginger, ground

Preparation:

Place the blackberries in a colander. Rinse well under cold running water and drain. Set aside.

Peel the kiwi and cut in half. Set aside.

Cut the cantaloupe in half. Scrape out the seeds and cut one one large wedge. Peel and chop into small pieces. Wrap the rest in a plastic foil and refrigerate for later.

Wash the apple and cut lengthwise in half. Remove the core and cut into bite-sized pieces. Set aside.

Now, combine cantaloupe, blackberries, kiwi, and apple in a juicer and process until juiced. Transfer to a serving glass and stir in the ginger.

Add few ice cubes and serve immediately.

Nutritional information per serving: Kcal: 181, Protein: 4.7g, Carbs: 56.3g, Fats: 1.6g

14.   Cucumber Strawberry Juice

Ingredients:

1 cup of cucumber, sliced

1 cup of strawberries, chopped

1 cup of blueberries

1 cup of fresh mint, torn

1 large carrot, sliced

¼ tsp of cinnamon, ground

Preparation:

Wash the cucumber and cut into thin slices. Fill the measuring cup and reserve the rest in the refrigerator.

Wash the strawberries and remove the stems. Chop into small pieces and set aside.

Wash the blueberries using a small colander. Drain and set aside.

Wash the mint thoroughly under cold running water. Drain and torn into small pieces. Set aside.

Wash and peel the carrot. Cut into thin slices and set aside.

Now, combine cucumber, strawberries, blueberries, mint, and carrot in a juicer. Process until well juiced.

Transfer to a serving glass and stir in the cinnamon. Add some crushed ice and serve immediately!

Nutrition information per serving: Kcal: 141, Protein: 4g, Carbs: 45g, Fats: 1.3g

15.   Honeydew Melon Watercress Juice

Ingredients:

1 large honeydew melon wedge

1 cup of watercress, torn

1 large artichoke

1 large green apple, cored

1 cup of mustard greens, torn

2 oz of water

¼ tsp of agave nectar

Preparation:

Cut the honeydew melon lengthwise in half. Scoop out the seeds using a spoon. Cut one large wedge and peel it. Cut into small chunks and place in a bowl. Wrap the rest of the melon in a plastic foil and refrigerate.

Combine watercress and mustard greens in a colander and wash under cold running water. Drain and set aside.

Trim off the outer leaves of the artichoke using a sharp knife. Cut into bite-sized pieces and set aside.

Wash the apple and remove the core. Cut into bite-sized pieces and set aside.

Now, process honeydew melon, watercress, artichoke, apple, and mustard greens in a juicer. Transfer to serving glasses and stir in the water and agave nectar.

Add some ice and serve immediately.

Nutritional information per serving: Kcal: 261, Protein: 9.4g, Carbs: 79.6g, Fats: 1.1g

16. Kale Orange Juice

Ingredients:

1 cup of kale, torn

1 large orange, peeled

1 cup of pineapple, chunked

1 cup of mango, chopped

1 small ginger knob, chopped

Preparation:

Wash the kale thoroughly under cold running water. Drain and torn into small pieces. Set aside.

Peel the orange and divide into wedges. Cut each wedge in half and set aside.

Using a sharp paring knife, cut the top of the pineapple. Gently remove all hard skin and cut it into small chunks. Fill the measuring cup and reserve the rest for later.

Peel the mango and chop into small pieces. Fill the measuring cup and reserve the rest for later. Set aside.

Peel the ginger knob and cut into small pieces. Set aside.

Now, combine pineapple, mango, kale, orange, and ginger in a juicer and process until juiced. Transfer to a serving glass and refrigerate for 15 minutes before serving.

Enjoy!

Nutrition information per serving: Kcal: 258, Protein: 6.9g, Carbs: 74.9g, Fats: 1.7g

17.   Tomato Basil Juice

Ingredients:

2 medium-sized Roma tomatoes, chopped

1 cup of fresh basil, torn

1 cup of pumpkin, cubed

1 large cucumber

¼ tsp of dried oregano

½ tsp of sea salt

2 oz of water

Preparation:

Wash the tomatoes and place them in a bowl. Cut into quarters and reserve the juice while cutting. Set aside.

Wash the basil thoroughly under cold running water. Torn with hands and set aside.

Peel the pumpkin and cut in half. Scoop out the seeds using a spoon. Cut one large wedge and peel it. Cut into small chunks and set aside. Reserve the rest for later.

Wash the cucumber and cut into thick slices. Set aside.

Now, process tomatoes, basil, pumpkin, and cucumber in a juicer. Transfer to serving glasses and stir in the oregano, salt, water, and reserved tomato juice.

Refrigerate for 5 minutes before serving.

Enjoy!

Nutritional information per serving: Kcal: 87, Protein: 4.9g, Carbs: 23.9g, Fats: 0.9g

18.   Peach Plum Juice

Ingredients:

1 large peach, chopped

1 whole plum, chopped

1 cup of mango, chopped

1 small Red Delicious apple, cored

1 oz of coconut water

Preparation:

Wash the peach and cut lengthwise in half. Remove the pit and cut into small pieces. Set aside.

Wash the plum and cut in half. Remove the pit and chop into small pieces. Set aside.

Peel the mango and cut into small cubes. Fill the measuring cup and reserve the rest for later.

Wash the apple cut lengthwise in half. Remove the core and chop into small pieces. Set aside.

Now, combine peach, plum, mango and apple in a juicer and process until juiced. Transfer to a serving glass and stir in the coconut water.

Add some ice and serve immediately.

Nutritional information per serving: Kcal: 252, Protein: 3.8g, Carbs: 71.1g, Fats: 1.6g

19.   Leek Beet Green Juice

Ingredients:

2 large leeks, chopped

1 cup of beet greens, torn

1 cup of broccoli

1 cup of arugula, torn

1 cup of collard greens, torn

1 large cucumber

1 large lime

A handful of spinach, torn

Preparation:

Wash the leeks and cut into small pieces. Set aside.

Combine arugula, beet greens, collard greens, and spinach in a colander. Wash under cold running water and torn with hands.

Wash the broccoli and cut into small chunks. Set aside.

Wash the cucumber and cut into thick slices. Set aside.

Peel the lime and cut lengthwise in half. Set aside.

Now, process arugula, beet greens, collard greens, spinach, leeks, broccoli, cucumber, and lime in a juicer. Transfer to serving glasses and refrigerate for 30 minutes before serving.

Enjoy!

Nutritional information per serving: Kcal: 194, Protein: 13.1g, Carbs: 55.7g, Fats: 1.8g

20.   Tomato Onion Juice

Ingredients:

1 medium-sized tomato, chopped

½ cup of spring onions, chopped

1 cup of cauliflower, chopped

½ cup of basil, torn

1 cup of cucumber, sliced

1 oz of water

Preparation:

Wash the tomato and place in a small bowl. Chop into small pieces and reserve the tomato juice while cutting. Set aside.

Wash the spring onions and basil. Chop into small pieces. Set aside.

Trim off the outer leaves of the cauliflower. Wash it and cut into small pieces. Fill the measuring cup and reserve the rest for later. Set aside.

Wash the cucumber and cut into thin slices. Fill the measuring cup and reserve the rest for later. Set aside.

Now, combine cauliflower, tomato, spring onions, basil, and cucumber in a juicer and process until well juiced. Transfer to a serving glass and stir in the water.

Serve cold.

Nutrition information per serving: Kcal: 51, Protein: 4.4g, Carbs: 13.9g, Fats: 0.7g

21.   Blueberry Zucchini Juice

Ingredients:

1 cup of blueberries

1 medium-sized zucchini, sliced

2 cups of raspberries

1 small ginger knob, peeled

1 oz of coconut water

Preparation:

Combine raspberries and blueberries in a large colander. Rinse well under cold running water. Drain and set aside.

Wash the zucchini and cut into thin slices. Set aside.

Peel the ginger knob and cut into small pieces. Set aside.

Now, combine raspberries, blueberries, zucchini, and ginger in a juicer and process until juiced. Transfer to a serving glass and stir in the coconut water.

Add crushed ice or refrigerate for 15 minutes before serving.

Enjoy!

Nutritional information per serving: Kcal: 164, Protein: 6.5g, Carbs: 58g, Fats: 2.7g

22. Swiss Chard Cauliflower Juice

Ingredients:

2 cups of Swiss chard

1 cup of cauliflower, chopped

3 large carrots, sliced

1 large lime, peeled

1 large orange, peeled

1 oz of water

Preparation:

Wash the Swiss chard thoroughly and torn with hands. Set aside.

Trim off the outer leaves of cauliflower. Wash it and cut into small pieces. Fill the measuring cup and reserve the rest in the refrigerator.

Wash the carrots and cut into thick slices. Set aside.

Peel the lime and cut lengthwise in half. Set aside.

Peel the orange and divide into wedges. Set aside.

Now, process carrots, Swiss chard, cauliflower, lime, and orange in a juicer. Transfer to serving glasses and stir in the water.

Add some ice and serve immediately.

Enjoy!

Nutritional information per serving: Kcal: 173, Protein: 7.3g, Carbs: 54g, Fats: 1.2g

23.   Raspberry Lemon Juice

Ingredients:

1 cup of raspberries

1 large lemon

1 large grapefruit

1 large lime

1 medium-sized yellow apple, cored

4oz of coconut water

Preparation:

Place the raspberries in a colander and wash under cold running water. Drain and set aside.

Peel the lemon and lime. Cut lengthwise in half and set aside.

Peel the grapefruit and divide into wedges. Set aside.

Wash the apple and remove the core. Cut into bite-sized pieces and set aside.

Now combine grapefruit, raspberries, lemon, lime, and apple in a juicer and process until juiced. Transfer to serving glasses and stir in the coconut water.

Add some ice and serve immediately.

Nutritional information per serving: Kcal: 240, Protein: 4.6g, Carbs: 76g, Fats: 1.6g

24.   Orange Spinach Juice

Ingredients:

1 large orange, peeled

½ cup of spinach, torn

1 cup of pineapple, chunked

3 Brussels sprouts, halved

Preparation:

Peel the orange and divide into wedges. Cut each wedge in half and set aside.

Wash the spinach thoroughly under cold running water and torn with hands. Set aside.

Using a sharp paring knife, cut the top of the pineapple. Gently remove all hard skin and slice it into thin slices. Fill the measuring cup and reserve the rest for later.

Wash the Brussels sprouts and trim off the wilted leaves. Cut each in half and set aside.

Now, combine orange, spinach, pineapple, and Brussels sprouts in a juicer and process until well juiced. Transfer to a serving glass and refrigerate for 15 minutes before serving.

Enjoy!

Nutrition information per serving: Kcal: 172, Protein: 7.9g, Carbs: 52.7g, Fats: 1.1g

25. Apple Ginger Juice

Ingredients:

1 small Golden Delicious apple, cored

¼ tsp of ginger, ground

1 cup of spinach, chopped

1 medium-sized wedge of honeydew melon

1 cup of raspberries

Preparation:

Wash the apple and cut lengthwise in half. Remove the core and cut into bite-sized pieces. Set aside.

Wash the spinach thoroughly under cold running water. Drain and chop into small pieces. Set aside.

Cut melon lengthwise in half. Scoop out the seeds and then wash the melon. Cut one wedge and peel it. Cut into bite-sized pieces and set aside. Reserve the rest in the refrigerator.

Place the raspberries in a colander and rinse well under cold running water. Drain and set aside.

Now, combine spinach, melon, raspberries, and apple in a juicer and process until juiced. Transfer to a serving glass and stir in the ginger. Add some ice before serving.

Enjoy!

Nutritional information per serving: Kcal: 142, Protein: 4.5g, Carbs: 46.1g, Fats: 1.4g

26. Pomegranate Orange Juice

Ingredients:

1 cup of pomegranate seeds

1 medium-sized orange, wedged

1 large pear, chopped

3 whole apricots, pitted

¼ tsp of cinnamon, ground

Preparation:

Cut the top of the pomegranate fruit using a sharp paring knife. Slice down to each of the white membranes inside of the fruit. Pop the seeds into a measuring cup and set aside.

Peel the orange and divide into wedges. Cut each wedge in half and set aside.

Wash the pear and cut lengthwise in half. Cut into bite-sized pieces and set aside.

Wash the apricots and cut each in half. Remove the pit and cut into small pieces. Set aside.

Now, combine pear, apricots, pomegranate seeds, and orange in a juicer. Process until well juiced. Transfer to a serving glass and stir in the cinnamon.

Refrigerate for 5 minutes before serving.

Nutrition information per serving: Kcal: 253, Protein: 4.9g, Carbs: 78.3g, Fats: 1.9g

27.   Celery Apple Juice

Ingredients:

1 cup of celery, chopped

1 medium-sized apple, cored

1 cup of sweet potatoes, cubed

1 medium-sized orange, peeled

1 tbsp of fresh mint, torn

Preparation:

Wash the celery and cut into bite-sized pieces. Set aside.

Wash the apple and cut lengthwise in half. Remove the core and cut into bite-sized pieces. Set aside.

Peel the sweet potato and cut into small cubes. Fill the measuring cup and reserve the rest for later. Set aside.

Peel the orange and divide into wedges. Cut each wedge in half and set aside.

Now, combine sweet potatoes, celery, apple, and orange in a juicer. Process until well juiced. Transfer to a serving glass and sprinkle with mint.

Add some crushed ice and serve immediately.

Nutrition information per serving: Kcal: 236, Protein: 4.7g, Carbs: 67.8g, Fats: 0.7g

28. Artichoke Cucumber Juice

Ingredients:

1 large artichoke, chopped

1 cup of cucumber, sliced

2 cups of Brussels sprouts, halved

¼ tsp of turmeric, ground

¼ tsp of ginger, ground

2 oz of water

Preparation:

Trim off the outer leaves of the artichoke. Cut into small pieces and set aside.

Wash the cucumber and cut into thin slices. Fill the measuring cup and reserve the rest in the refrigerator.

Wash the Brussels sprouts and trim off the outer layers. Cut each sprout in half and fill the measuring cups. Set aside.

Now, combine Brussels sprouts, artichoke, and cucumber in a juicer and process until well juiced. Transfer to a serving glass and stir in the ginger, turmeric, and water.

Refrigerate for 15 minutes before serving.

Enjoy!

Nutritional information per serving: Kcal: 98, Protein: 11.6g, Carbs: 34.7g, Fats: 0.8g

29.   Banana Strawberry Juice

Ingredients:

1 large banana, sliced

½ cup of strawberries, chopped

1 cup of avocado, chunked

1 cup of red leaf lettuce, shredded

1 small Red Delicious apple, cored

¼ tsp of cinnamon, ground

Preparation:

Peel the banana and chop into small pieces. Set aside.

Wash the strawberries and remove the stems. Cut into bite-sized pieces and fill the measuring cup. Set aside.

Peel the avocado and cut lengthwise in half. Remove the pit and chop into small pieces. Set aside.

Wash the lettuce thoroughly under cold running water. Drain and chop into small pieces. Set aside.

Now, combine avocado, lettuce, banana, and strawberries in a juicer and process until juiced. Transfer to a serving glass and stir in the cinnamon.

Add some ice and serve immediately.

Enjoy!

Nutritional information per serving: Kcal: 405, Protein: 5.7g, Carbs: 72.2g, Fats: 23.1g

30.   Basil Cucumber Juice

Ingredients:

1 cup of fresh basil, torn

1 cup of cucumber, sliced

1 cup of celery, chopped

1 whole lime, peeled

1 medium-sized apple, cored

Preparation:

Wash the basil thoroughly under cold running water. Drain and torn into small pieces. Set aside.

Wash the cucumber and cut into thin slices. Fill the measuring cup and reserve the rest for later. Set aside.

Wash the celery and cut into small pieces. Set aside.

Peel the lime and cut lengthwise in half. Set aside.

Wash the apple and cut lengthwise in half. Remove the core and cut into bite-sized pieces. Set aside.

Now, combine celery, basil, cucumber, lime, and apple in a juicer and process until well juiced. Transfer to a serving glass and add some crushed ice.

Serve immediately.

Nutritional information per serving: Kcal: 109, Protein: 2.7g, Carbs: 31.9g, Fats: 0.7g

31.   Orange Cantaloupe Juice

Ingredients:

1 large orange

1 cup of cantaloupe

1 cup of strawberries

1 large carrot

2 oz of water

Preparation:

Peel the orange and divide into wedges. Set aside.

Cut the cantaloupe in half. Scoop out the seeds. Cut two wedges and peel them. Chop into chunks and set aside. Reserve the rest of the cantaloupe in a refrigerator.

Wash the strawberries under cold running water. Drain and cut in half. Set aside.

Wash the carrot and cut into thick slices. Set aside.

Now, combine strawberries, orange, cantaloupe, and carrot in a juicer and process until juiced.

Transfer to serving glasses and stir in the water. Add some ice and serve immediately.

Nutritional information per serving: Kcal: 177, Protein: 4.9g, Carbs: 55g, Fats: 1.2g

32.   Apple Pomegranate Juice

Ingredients:

1 large red apple, cored

1 cup of pomegranate seeds

2 large beets, trimmed

1 large cucumber

1 small ginger knob, 1-inch

Preparation:

Wash the apple and remove the core. Cut into bite-sized pieces and set aside.

Cut the top of the pomegranate fruit using a sharp knife. Slice down to each of the white membranes inside of the fruit. Pop the seeds into a medium bowl.

Wash the beets and trim off the green parts. Cut into small pieces and set aside.

Wash the cucumber and cut into thick slices. Set aside.

Peel the ginger knob and set aside.

Now, process beets, apple, pomegranate seeds, cucumber and ginger knob in a juicer. Transfer to serving glasses and add some ice. You can stir in one tablespoon of honey, but this is optional.

Serve immediately.

Nutritional information per serving: Kcal: 285, Protein: 8g, Carbs: 81.6g, Fats: 2.2g

33.   Collard Green Cucumber Juice

Ingredients:

1 cup of collard greens, chopped

1 cup of cucumber, sliced

1 whole fennel bulb, chopped

1 whole lemon, peeled

1 oz of water

¼ tsp of cayenne pepper, ground

Preparation:

Rinse the collard greens under cold running water. Drain and chop into small pieces. Set aside.

Wash the cucumber and cut into thin slices. Fill the measuring cup and reserve the rest for later. Set aside.

Trim off the fennel bulb and remove the green parts. Wash the bulb and cut into small pieces. Set aside.

Peel the lemon and cut lengthwise in half. Set aside.

Now, combine fennel, collard greens, cucumber, and lemon in a juicer and process until juiced. Transfer to a serving glass and stir in the water and cayenne pepper.

Refrigerate for 20 minutes before serving.

Enjoy!

Nutritional information per serving: Kcal: 68, Protein: 4.9g, Carbs: 26.3g, Fats: 0.9g

34.   Apple Strawberry Juice

Ingredients:

1 small green apple, cored

1 cup of strawberries, chopped

1 cup of cherries, pitted

2 whole plums, pitted and chopped

1 tbsp of coconut water

¼ tsp of ginger, ground

Preparation:

Wash the apple and cut lengthwise in half. Remove the core and cut into small pieces. Set aside.

Wash the strawberries and remove the stems. Cut into small pieces and fill the measuring cup. Reserve the rest for later. Set aside.

Wash the cherries thoroughly using a large colander. Drain and cut each in half. Remove the pits and cut into small pieces. Set aside.

Wash the plums and cut in half. Remove the pits and cut into small bite-sized pieces. Set aside.

Now, combine apple, strawberries, cherries, and plums in a juicer and process until juiced. Transfer to a serving glass and stir in the coconut water and ginger.

Add some crushed ice and serve immediately.

Nutritional information per serving: Kcal: 236, Protein: 4.2g, Carbs: 70.3g, Fats: 1.3g

35.   Cabbage Avocado Juice

Ingredients:

1 cup of green cabbage, torn

1 cup of avocado, cubed

1 large artichoke, chopped

1 cup of fresh spinach, torn

¼ tsp of turmeric, ground

Preparation:

Combine spinach and cabbage in a large colander. Wash thoroughly under cold running water. Drain and torn into small pieces. Set aside.

Peel the avocado and cut lengthwise in half. Remove the pit and cut into small cubes. Fill the measuring cup and reserve the rest in the refrigerator.

Trim off the outer layers of the artichoke using a sharp paring knife. Cut into bite-sized pieces and set aside.

Now, combine artichoke, spinach, cabbage, and avocado in a juicer and process until juiced. Transfer to a serving glass and stir in the turmeric.

Refrigerate for 10 minutes before serving.

Nutritional information per serving: Kcal: 282, Protein: 15.4g, Carbs: 42.6g, Fats: 23.2g

36.   Avocado Cantaloupe Juice

Ingredients:

1 cup of avocado chunks

1 cup of cantaloupe, chopped

3 cups of celery, chopped

1 cup of fresh basil, torn

1 cup of cucumber, sliced

2 oz of water

Preparation:

Peel the avocado and cut in half. Remove the pit and cut into chunks. Fill the measuring cup and refrigerate the rest for some other juice.

Cut the cantaloupe in half. Scoop out the seeds and flesh. Cut two wedges and peel them. Chop into chunks and set aside. Reserve the rest of the cantaloupe in a refrigerator.

Wash the celery and cut into small pieces. Set aside.

Wash the basil thoroughly under cold running water. Drain and torn with hands. Set aside.

Wash the cucumber and cut into thick slices. Set aside.

Now, process avocado, cantaloupe, celery, basil, and cucumber in a juicer. Transfer to serving glasses and refrigerate for 15 minutes before serving.

Enjoy!

Nutritional information per serving: Kcal: 288, Protein: 7.5g, Carbs: 37.1g, Fats: 23g

37.   Melon Carrot Juice

Ingredients:

1 large honeydew melon wedge

2 large carrots

1 large artichoke

1 large grapefruit

1 small ginger root knob, 1-inch

2 oz of water

Preparation:

Cut the honeydew melon lengthwise in half. Scoop out the seeds using a spoon. Cut a large wedge and peel it. Cut into small chunks and place in a bowl. Wrap the rest of the melon in a plastic foil and refrigerate.

Wash the carrots and cut into thick slices. Set aside.

Using a sharp knife, trim off the outer wilted layers of artichoke. Cut into small chunks and set aside.

Peel the grapefruit and divide into wedges. Set aside.

Peel the ginger knob and set aside.

Now, process, artichoke, grapefruit, honeydew melon, carrots, and ginger in a juicer.

Transfer to serving glasses and stir in the water. Add some ice and serve immediately.

Enjoy!

Nutritional information per serving: Kcal: 230, Protein: 9.5g, Carbs: 72.6g, Fats: 1.1g

38.   Apple Lime Juice

Ingredients:

1 large green apple, cored

1 large lime, peeled

1 cup of mango chunks

1 large orange, peeled

1 small ginger root knob, 1-inch

2 oz of water

Preparation:

Wash the apple and remove the core. Cut into bite-sized pieces and set aside.

Peel the lime and cut lengthwise in half. Set aside.

Wash the mango and cut into chunks. Fill the measuring cup and refrigerate the rest for some other juice.

Peel the orange and divide into wedges. Set aside.

Peel the ginger knob and set aside.

Now, process mango, orange, apple, lime, and ginger in a juicer. Transfer to serving glasses and stir in the water.

Add some ice and serve immediately.

Enjoy!

Nutritional information per serving: Kcal: 268, Protein: 12.8g, Carbs: 53g, Fats: 1.5g

39. Kale Lettuce Juice

Ingredients:

1 cup of kale, torn

1 cup Romaine lettuce, torn

1 cup of crookneck squash

1 cup of collard greens,torn

1 large cucumber

½ tsp of Himalayan salt

¼ tsp of Cayenne pepper, ground

2 oz of water

Preparation:

Combine collard greens, kale, and lettuce in a colander. Wash thoroughly under cold running water and torn with hands. Set aside.

Wash the crookneck squash and cut in half. Scoop out the seeds using a spoon. Cut into small chunks and set aside. Reserve the rest for another juice.

Wash the cucumber and chop into thick slices. Set aside.

Now, combine crookneck squash, collard greens, kale, lettuce, and cucumber ina juicer and process until juiced.

Transfer to serving glasses and stir in the salt, Cayenne pepper, and water. Refrigerate for 15 minutes before serving.

Nutritional information per serving: Kcal: 91, Protein: 7.8g, Carbs: 25.2g, Fats: 1.6g

ADDITIONAL TITLES FROM THIS AUTHOR

70 Effective Meal Recipes to Prevent and Solve Being Overweight: Burn Fat Fast by Using Proper Dieting and Smart Nutrition

By

Joe Correa CSN

48 Acne Solving Meal Recipes: The Fast and Natural Path to Fixing Your Acne Problems in Less Than 10 Days!

By

Joe Correa CSN

41 Alzheimer's Preventing Meal Recipes: Reduce or Eliminate Your Alzheimer's Condition in 30 Days or Less!

By

Joe Correa CSN

70 Effective Breast Cancer Meal Recipes: Prevent and Fight Breast Cancer with Smart Nutrition and Powerful Foods

By

Joe Correa CSN

www.ingramcontent.com/pod-product-compliance
Lightning Source LLC
Chambersburg PA
CBHW030300030426
42336CB00009B/463